BE BETTER

Copyright © 2025 by Jennifer Chen
All rights reserved. No part of this book may be reproduced in any manner whatsoever without written permission except in the case of brief quotations embodied in critical articles and reviews.
First Printing, 2025

Be Better

Jennifer Chen

Dedicated to

My family, who love, support,
and believe in me.
My friends, who help me through
everything life brings.
My clients, who trust me with their health
and encouraged me to share this.
And to you, because you deserve to
live better and be better.

Contents

A Small Change Everyday Day   vii

Part One   1
  1 Posture Checks   2
  2 Ankle Alphabet   8
  3 Toe Stretches and Ankle Circles   12
  4 Toe Grab and Push   15
  5 Agility Training   18
  6 Stretch   22
  7 Balance   26
  8 Cat Cow / Bird Dog   31
  9 Practice Big Steps   36
 10 Keep On Stepping   40
 11 Tongue Training   44

Part Two   47
 12 Food Log   48
 13 Buy the Rainbow, Eat the Rainbow   58

14	Eat This First	62
15	Half a Plateful of Fruits and Veggies	65
16	Salad Plate	69
17	Drink Your Water	72
Part Three		76
18	Three Kind Choices	77
19	Reach Out	80
20	Meditate	83
21	Sunshine and Sunscreen	87
22	Try Something New	90
23	Read	94
24	Put Down the Screens	97
25	Dance Party	100
26	Be Thankful	103

About the Author   106

A Small Change Everyday Day

How can you start living a healthier life? The answer is simple, just make one or two minor changes a day. Each of these slight changes, with practice, leads to bigger, life altering changes. Whether assessing your posture, eating a little better each day to establish a healthier routine, or stretching your body, it all comes down to making a small change each day.

Big changes often feel unobtainable, overwhelming, or can lead to burnout. Instead, I offer ideas to Be Better just a little, every day. By continuing to incorporate these changes each day, it can lead to healthier outcomes for your future.

So, how does this book work? I challenge you to read one or two lessons (chapters) every week. Then incorporate the homework described each day for a week. Each chapter states the homework, lists considerations or equipment needed, offers instructions to complete the homework, and lists some of the benefits.

Before starting any new fitness routine or diet, please consult your doctor. The homework provided is for the general population and may or may not apply to you. If you have any questions or concerns about how any of these chapters can impact you, please consult your medical professional for further guidance.

Included in this book are lessons to improve your agility, balance, coordination, flexibility, and core strength and stability. There are lessons aimed at decreasing foot, back, and neck pain. Other lessons develop skills to maintain a healthier diet, practice mindfulness, and create a more loving community.

The first lesson to read is Posture Checks. This chapter teaches you how to get into good posture which is needed to perform several other chapters safely and effectively. Then, you are more than welcome to skip around and practice whichever you choose. I typically give one or two lessons (homeworks) a week, mixing and matching from each section to give variety. I suggest reading the For the Belly section in order, as the information builds.

These small homework assignments have impacted me and my clients. After I gave the homework of "Try Something New," my clients encouraged me to write this book in the hopes that I could influence you to try new things to help improve your life.

You can Be Better by starting with a small change every day.

In health and wellness,
Jen

Part One

FOR THE BODY

"A strong body is the foundation of all happiness." - Leigh Hunt

"Take care of your body. It's the only place you have to live." – Jim Rohn

"Exercise not only changes your body, it changes your mind, your attitude, and your mood." – Unknown

1

Posture Checks

> *Your homework everyday this week is to practice three "posture checks."*

How to do your homework: If you are seated, adjust the height of the chair so your feet rest flat on the floor, your knees should be below the level of your hips. Try to keep your pelvis steady and neutral. If you have a back support or pillow, place it behind the low back. Engage your core and lift your ribcage, try to create as much distance as possible from your ribcage to your pelvis. Bring your shoulders down and back. Your ears should be above your shoulders.

If you are standing, to get into a proper posture, you want to stand with your feet hip distance apart. Your knees should have a slight bend and be over your ankles, hips over your knees, neutral pelvis and core engaged, shoulders over the hips (making sure to draw them down and back), and your ears should be over your shoulders.

Now that we are in good posture, take a deep breath in and ask yourself, "Does my neck feel stiff?" Very slowly nodding your head to answer, "yes."

Again, ask yourself, "Does my neck still feel stiff?" Slowly bring your ear to each shoulder, to reply "I don't know." It is important to do this slowly and not to lift up the shoulders.

Finally, ask yourself again, "Does my neck still feel stiff?" This time, slowly turn your head side to side to say, "not anymore."

Next, say "Whoooohooo!" as you do slow neck circles in each direction.

Let's take a second to do it together right now. Regardless of whether you are sitting or standing, take a moment to get into the proper posture. Take a deep breath and ask yourself, "does my neck feel stiff?" Lift your chin up and bring your chin down, while answering "yes it does." Ask yourself again, bringing your ear towards your shoulder on your exhale, answering, "I don't know." Make sure to go slow and within your range of motion. One last time, ask yourself, "does my neck still feel stiff?" slowly turn your head to say, "not anymore." Lastly, say "whooooohooo," while doing a neck circle in each direction.

How does this help you Be Better?

The benefits of maintaining the proper posture are far reaching. The most noticeable benefits are the physical ones, but there are psychological benefits as well.

People with good posture are less likely to suffer from back and neck pain. This occurs because keeping the spine in good alignment reduces the stress on the spine. Poor posture affects the muscles, bones, ligaments, and the nerves of the neck and spine, leading to muscle imbalances and worse posture. When our body tries to adjust for the imbalance, it creates instability or misalignment. Staying in good posture decreases the risk of injury, especially chronic back pain, and neck injury.

Maintaining the correct posture forces the body to engage the muscles in the core to stabilize the spine, increasing core and postural muscle strength. This also has an added benefit of improving balance.

A condition with correlations to posture is tension headaches. While there is no single cause of tension headaches, they can be triggered by poor posture. Partly because our nervous system runs down the spine and partly because there is added weight to the back of the neck and shoulders. By bringing the shoulders down and back, it lessens the stress placed on the base of the neck, the spot we carry our tension. This decreases the likelihood of tension headaches.

Our posture affects digestion by either compressing or decompressing the organs and nerves of the digestive tract. In bad posture, our digestive system does not have enough space and is compressed. When the digestive tract is compressed, the nerves cannot communicate as effectively with the digestive organs to move waste. Unfortunately, this makes the digestive system less efficient. In good posture, the digestive tract is decompressed, and our nerves can tell our organs to move waste along. This allows better movement of waste through the body.

Lung capacity is improved when we are in good posture. This happens because our posture dictates how much space the intercostal muscles and diaphragm can expand during breath. Good posture allows the lungs to expand fully and bring in full breaths. This means more oxygen for the body and brain.

When the body gets enough oxygen, it leads to "happier" muscles. When the brain gets enough oxygen, it leads to better overall mental wellbeing. More oxygen to the brain has been shown to benefit mood and cognitive function. Moreover, there have been multiple studies in which participants self-reported feeling more confident and optimistic, and less fearful while in good posture.

Unfortunately, due to the use of electronic devices, maintaining the proper posture has been increasingly difficult. Tech (or Text) Neck Syndrome is a syndrome caused by the repetitive weight of leaning forward to look at devices for prolonged periods of time.

The human head weighs between ten to twelve pounds and is supported by the neck. The neck is comprised of seven bones called the cervical vertebrae. Between each vertebra there is a shock absorbing intervertebral disc. The vertebrae are surrounded by muscles, tendons, ligaments, and nerves. These are the structures that support and move our head.

Depending on the degree in which we lean forward to look at our devices, it can add undue force onto your neck. The further forward we lean, the more weight is added to our neck and spinal muscles and the more damage we do to the cervical vertebrae.

In 2014, orthopedic and spinal surgeon Dr. Kenneth Hansraj published the <u>Assessment of Stresses in the Cervical Spine Caused by Posture and Position of the Head</u> in the National Library of Medicine. In the research presented, the further forward your head tilts, the more weight and pressure is put on your spine. Tilting the head fifteen degrees forward places roughly twenty-seven pounds of pressure on your cervical spine; tilting your head forward by forty-five degrees places forty-nine pounds of pressure on the cervical spine; and tilting sixty degrees forward places sixty pounds of pressure on the cervical spine.

There are simple things that can improve your back and neck health if you are using devices. One way is to position your devices so you do not have to tilt your head down. Another is to take frequent breaks to stretch your back and reestablish your posture.

And the best way to reestablish proper posture is with a posture check. In the time it took to read the last few paragraphs, have your shoulders slumped? Are your ears over your shoulders? Is your core still engaged?

Let's go ahead and do another posture check while we are here. Take a deep breath in, settle your feet, engage your core, think tall thoughts, bring those shoulders down and back, and lift your chin. Does your neck feel stiff? Answer with, "Yes," "I don't know," "no," and "whooooohoooo!" Now, put your hands on your hips and remind yourself, "I am a superhuman. I got this!"

By my count, you have done at least two posture checks for the day, which means you only need to do one more to finish your homework! If you would like bonus points for this week's homework, do a posture check or two while using your phone, computer, or tablet.

I hope this lesson and homework leaves you feeling more confident and optimistic.

2

Ankle Alphabet

Your homework everyday this week is to write each of the letters of the alphabet with each foot.

Considerations: Though this is an ankle rehabilitation exercise, this is not meant to treat or cure foot or ankle injury. If you have ankle pain or injury, consult your medical provider first. If these stretches cause pain, stop.

How to do your homework: this homework can be done while lying, sitting, or standing. If lying, put a pillow or rolled up towel underneath your working leg's calf. If sitting or standing, get in good posture, lifting your working leg three to four inches and using something to hold on to, if needed. While keeping the working leg still, use your foot to write each letter of the alphabet from A-Z while only moving the ankle. Switch to the other side. If you need to switch feet every few letters or take breaks, then go ahead.

As you progress, you can make your letters bigger and add additional sets. Recommendations vary by physical and physiotherapists. Some recommend one to three sets a day, some say more if there is no pain. Some say uppercase, or lowercase, others say both.

That said, you know your body. Start with one set, go slowly and deliberately. This is a lot harder than it seems, if you are pain free and want to progress, consider doing another set. As always, contact your provider if you experience any pain or have any questions.

How does this help you Be Better?

The benefits of the ankle alphabet exercise include building ankle strength, flexibility, and stability while decreasing risk of falls.

While writing every letter of the alphabet, your ankle is flexing, extending, everting, and inverting. Over time, this exercise addresses weak ankles by strengthening the muscles, bones, ligaments, and tendons that support the ankle. When we continue to practice this, we also increase the flexibility and ease of movement of the ankle.

Strong and flexible muscles are happy muscles. Strengthening the muscles around the ankles has been shown to prevent injuries by reducing pressure on the ankle joint and increasing the surrounding bone density. Flexibility around the ankle aids in recovery time in ankle injuries.

Ankle strengthening and increase in range of motion improves stability. Improved stability and flexibility of the ankle decreases the risk of falls and improves balance. This occurs because when our ground becomes unstable, one of the first things our body does to regain balance is to stabilize our ankles. If our ankles are weak or inflexible, we are less likely to regain our balance.

I was out on a walk with one of my aunts and we were talking about the homework I give my clients, and she suggested this as a potential homework assignment. My aunt told me after she sprained her ankle decades ago, her medical provider suggested this to her. She appreciated this homework so much that it stuck with her.

After our conversation, I researched the Ankle Alphabet and started doing it on my own. Soon after, it was added to the homework rotation. Now, it is a client favorite.

So, let's do this together. If lying, put a pillow or towel under your leg. If seated or standing, get into good posture (ears over shoulders, think tall thoughts, hips neutral and under the shoulders), and grab onto something, if needed. Lift your working leg and by only moving your ankle, write the letters A-M of the alphabet, all upper case. Switch to the other side and repeat. Continue by finishing the alphabet N-Z on each side. If you would like, you can repeat this.

Excellent job! Your goal is to do this every day this week. You got this!

PS My favorite place to do this is in bed. I do it when I wake up to prepare my feet for the day, and before I go to bed after an exhausting day.

3

Toe Stretches and Ankle Circles

> *Your homework everyday this week is to stretch your toes by toe splaying and dorsiflexion, then to do ankle rotations.*

How to do your homework: Sit down in good posture; ears over shoulders, shoulders down and back, neutral pelvis, and core engaged. Have your bare feet resting on the floor. While keeping the heels and balls of the feet pressed into the ground, lift the toes off the ground and try to stretch your toes as far apart as possible. This is called splaying your toes. It is important not to strain or hold your breath. Hold for 2 to 3 breaths then relax your feet. Try for six to eight repetitions.

Next, do another posture check. Cross an ankle over the shin or knee. Gently pull the toes towards the shin, this is called dorsiflexion. Hold for 2 to 3 breaths. Repeat if you want. Next, roll your ankle into five big circles in each direction. Repeat, including the posture check, on the other side.

How does this help you Be Better?

Splaying the toes maintains foot alignment, increases flexibility of the toes, and improves stability and balance. Pulling the toes towards the shin aids with stretching the muscles that contract the toes. Lastly, ankle rotations benefit ankle flexibility, strength, and balance.

Splaying the toes helps maintain strong feet and proper foot alignment. When the toes can spread properly, it helps disperse pressure through the foot. This helps keep the foot and toes better aligned. When our toes and feet are misaligned, it can lead to joint pain, muscle imbalances, muscle overcompensation, and strains on other parts of the body. Splaying the toes increases circulation and blood flow to the feet while decreasing toe and foot stiffness. This may reduce foot pain, cramps, and plantar fasciitis.

An important function of the toes is to help maintain balance during movement by gripping onto the ground. Regularly splaying the toes increases the range of motion and strength of the toes while reducing pain and stiffness. These benefits allow the toes to better spread and grip the ground providing more stability.

Ankle rotations keep the ankle joint flexible. This flexibility allows the foot to better stabilize on uneven surfaces. Flexibility and mobility of the ankle makes everyday activities like walking, squatting, and changing direction more efficient as well as less stressful on your body's joints. Stiff ankles can lead to muscle imbalances in the knees, hips, and lower back.

Ankle rotation strengthens the muscles around the ankle joint. By building the muscles surrounding the ankle joint it reduces the pressure on the ankle joint and increases bone density. This can help prevent injury. Strengthening these muscles, ligaments, and tendons also improves the proprioceptors (sensory receptors that relay body positioning) on the feet, aiding in stabilization and fall prevention.

Keeping your toes, feet, and ankles strong and flexible is paramount to maintaining the ability to walk, stand, reach, and sidestep. Our feet absorb the pressures of our weight and our movements, so it is important that we take great care of them. Think about how much our feet support us on a day-to-day basis. Therefore, it is important to add foot care to our daily routine.

Let's take a moment to help our feet relax. Take your shoes off, sit up nice and tall, keep your heels on the ground, lift and spread your toes out as far as you can. Hold the stretch for 2-3 breaths and release. When you are ready, cross one ankle over your knee or shin bone and interlace your fingers through your toes. If you cannot, that's fine. Gently pull your toes toward the shin. Then rotate your ankle in both directions. Take a deep breath and switch sides.

Great job in completing your homework! Be sure to try this after a long day. Your feet will thank you!

4

Toe Grab and Push

> *Your homework everyday this week is to use your toes to pull a hand or dish towel toward you, then use your toes to push the towel away.*

How to do your homework: While seated, lay the towel flat on the floor and step onto the towel so your heels are at the bottom. Next, do a posture check. Make sure your feet are resting flat on the floor, keeping your pelvis steady and neutral, engaging your core, and bringing your shoulders down and back. Your ears should be above your shoulders. Ask yourself, "does my neck feel stiff?" (Yes, I don't know, no, and whoooohooo).

To get the most out of this exercise, make sure your heels are firmly on the ground. Now, slowly pull the towel with your toes. Flex (curl) your toes and pull the towel towards you. After bringing the towel all the way, use your toes to push the towel all the way away from you. Opinions differ with how many of these to do. Start with two to three repetitions and add slowly if you choose.

How does this help you Be Better?

The benefits of flexing and curling your toes include stronger toes, better shock absorption, flexibility and stability, which all contribute to better balance.

The pulling and pushing motion in this exercise helps improve the strength in the muscles that contract our toes. Strong toe muscles provide better support for your body weight and better absorb the impact of daily activities. It also improves the circulation and range of motion of the muscles, tendons, and ligaments of the feet. By improving the range of motion, it reduces foot stiffness and may help prevent common foot injuries like Achilles tendinitis and plantar fasciitis. It also leads to improvements in agility, power, and speed.

Flexibility in the toes aids in the stability of the toes and feet. Toe stability helps with leaning forward without falling. As you get older, toe stability and toe strength lessen, leading to possible forward leaning falls. By practicing this exercise, it improves a person's Toe Grip Strength (TGS), which is the ability for the toes to grab onto the floor to stabilize yourself. TGS can help prevent falls and help in the process of standing. Research shows that people with lower TGS are at a higher risk for falls.

Toe strength and flexibility are important aspects of walking, balance, and fall prevention. This simple exercise helps build strength and flexibility and should be added as a rehabilitation or as part of a warmup to a workout. Always remember to add repetitions slowly and carefully.

If you haven't already, grab a towel, sit tall in a chair, and let's do this!

5

Agility Training

> *Your homework everyday this week is to practice your agility by taking a few steps side to side and a few steps forward and backward.*

Considerations: Agility training is training your body to change your direction, speed, and body positioning safely and effectively. If you are new to fitness, have balance, gait, or mobility issues, consider doing agility training in front of a mirror or next to a table or wall to assist with balance. Also, make sure the area in which you are practicing is free from obstacles or hazards. Most importantly, work within your range of motion and your comfort. You decide what feels good for you and what works well for you. As always, start small and build your skills before progressing.

How to do this homework: Before doing this homework, assess where you are. Are there any obstacles or tripping hazards? If so, remove them. Only when your practice area is safe should you continue.

From here, take a deep breath and get into good posture: ears over the shoulders, shoulders down and back, creating space between the shoulders and the hips, core engaged, knees soft and under your hips. Now, take four small steps to the right. Step, together, step, together, step, together, step, together. Now, four small steps to the left. One more time, each way. If you feel safe, progress to medium sized steps. Four to the right, then four to the left. Next, take four steps forward and four steps back. And repeat.

Only step as quickly and as largely as you feel comfortable and confident in doing. If needed, hold onto something or widen your stance to assist with balance.

If you are ready to progress, you can shuffle, take larger steps, or make it a grapevine. Other progressions for agility training include adding exercises such as heel kicks, high knees, or squats. You can continue to progress by adding weight or increasing the range of motion or speed in your steps. If you want, do your agility training while listening to music.

There are videos online showing several types of agility training and progressions when you are ready. Make sure to use accredited sources. Again, only progress if you can safely do so.

How does this help you Be Better?

Agility training is one of the most important things you can do to keep your body safe as you get older. Agility training strengthens multiple groups of muscles, increases body awareness, builds core stability and balance.

Agility training strengthens the muscles, ligaments, bones, and tendons surrounding the knee, ankle, and foot. This helps slow the natural weakening of those muscles as you age and may aid in shorter recovery times after a workout.

This training also teaches the body to maintain balance between the top half and the bottom half while the body is in motion. This increases body awareness, coordination, and balance while building muscle memory. As body awareness, coordination, and balance improve, the risk of fall and fall related injury decreases.

This is one of the most important homework challenges that you can do. By consistently practicing moving sideways, forward, and back, we teach our body how to move in those directions safely. As we age, we take less backward and sideways steps, getting less practice. This increases the chance of falling in those directions. By practicing walking in all directions, it may lead to being able to catch ourselves if we start to fall in those directions, helping avoid falls and the injuries that come with falls.

I had this client, an older gentleman, who scoffed at the homework during class and seemed not to care in front of me. Little did I know, he did his homework regularly. One day he caught himself falling and was able to stabilize himself, preventing a fall. He later confided that he thought he was able to catch himself because of all the agility training he did.

It is my hope that your agility training will help you too.

> "If you want to maintain your ability,
> to keep your stability,
> then practice your agility."
> – Jennifer Chen

6

Stretch

> *Your homework everyday this week is to stretch for at least ten minutes each day.*

Considerations: Stretching should not cause pain. If you are stretching past your range of motion, you can and will hurt yourself. If you are stretching in bad form, you can hurt yourself. If you are holding your breath while stretching, you can hurt yourself.

How to do your homework: There are three types of stretching: dynamic, static, and ballistic. Dynamic stretches are movement-based stretches that can improve agility and coordination. Most dynamic stretching is done as a warmup as a gentle pre-workout, loosening up the muscles which you will use during the workout.

Static stretches are held stretches that relax the muscles to increase range of motion. These stretches are held for about fifteen to thirty seconds at the end of your workout. Stretching the muscles you already have used. If you want to deepen a static stretch, prepare on your inhale and extend on your exhale making sure to control your movements.

The last type is ballistic stretching. Ballistic stretching CAN CAUSE INJURY and IS NOT RECOMMENDED. Ballistic stretching occurs when a force, like momentum, is used to stretch past the normal range of motion. This leads to uncontrolled, jerky, or bouncy stretches. An example of this is bouncing when trying to touch and reach your toes. This stretching is not controlled and therefore can lead to muscle imbalance and tears.

According to the National Academy of Sports Medicine (NASM), ideally, people should stretch each major muscle and tendon group everyday but at a minimum of two to three times a week. In terms of static stretches, NASM suggests holding each stretch for 15-60 seconds, and stretching to the point of tightness (not pain or discomfort).

If stretching is not something you do regularly, start small. I recommend stretching in front of a mirror so you can make sure you are in good form. If you need inspiration, look up "beginner stretch guide" videos first and make sure to use a trusted source.

How does this help you Be Better?

Stretching is the best way to maintain happy muscles and joints, increase range of motion, and help relax.

Proper stretching releases tight muscles which can improve aches and pains, stress, circulation, and posture.

Stretching decreases the risk of injury by reducing muscle and joint stiffness while improving range of motion and muscle strength. This improves recovery outcomes and helps alleviate the muscle fatigue that comes with day-to-day activities.

Flexibility in the joints and muscles allows more ease and efficiency in daily movements. Further, stretching helps maintain your range of motion. As you age, your range of motion decreases. Stretching regularly helps maintain and may improve your range of motion.

The best part of stretching (in my opinion) is feeling calm. Stretching gives a person time to relax and become self-aware with their body. Studies have linked daily stretching to reduced anxiety and stress, and with better focus and sleep. This occurs because our body releases serotonin and endorphins when we stretch, boosting our mood and aiding in relaxation.

Consider all the movements we make every day. All the stress we inadvertently place on our body. It is important that we take the time, even if it is just a few minutes here and there, to stretch. It helps keep the muscles, bones, and joints healthy. Stretching calms the mind while it relaxes the body.

Every class, I ask my clients if they are ready for my "favorite part of the day," and then we stretch. It is the time when we get to relax our body and the muscles we have used. It is my time to be thankful for all my body has allowed me to accomplish.

So, if you are ready to, let's start stretching! Again, make sure to stay in proper form, breathe deep, and go slow. Hopefully, stretching will become your favorite part of the day as well.

7

Balance

> *Your homework everyday this week is to practice and challenge your balance every day.*

Considerations: If you have balance, gait, or mobility issues, then I recommend starting in a shallow water pool (bust to armpit level water) and then progressing to land. Again, make sure to start small and build your skills before progressing.

If you are progressing to land, consider practicing in front of a mirror, with someone to help you, or next to something to hold onto (like a chair) to assist your balance. The safest place on land to practice is with your back to a walled corner, with a chair and mirror in front of you.

Your practice area should be free from obstacles or hazards. Most importantly, do not progress until you feel safe to do so. You decide what feels good for you and what works well for you.

How to do your homework: It is important to maintain good posture throughout this homework. So please take a moment and do a posture check. Ears over shoulders, core engaged, pelvis neutral, ankles and knees under the hips. Considering how everybody and every body is different; everyone will start at different places for this homework.

Lower body progressions for balance:

First, start with a wide stance, bringing the feet a little wider than hip distance apart. The wider your stance, the wider your base of support and the more balanced you will feel. If needed, bend your knees to lower your center of gravity, and make you feel more stable. If you feel safe, you can bring your feet hip width apart, and progress to bringing your feet together, and then to your feet touching.

If you would like to continue, step one foot back into a tandem stance. If this is challenging, widen the tandem stance, if this is not challenging enough, bring your stance narrower. You can progress into a tightrope stance (one foot directly behind the other like on a tightrope). Make sure you practice slowly and on both sides. If you are ready, the next progression is a one-legged stance.

If you would like to further challenge your balance, you can do so by standing or balancing on an unstable surface. The unstable surface forces the body to make small adjustments to stabilize the foot. These small adjustments take place because the body's proprioceptors (sensory receptors that relay body positioning) sense an uneven ground and work to stabilize. This training is called proprioceptive training and has been shown to better aid agility, motor function, and balance. Ankle proprioception plays an essential role in balance, reaction time, coordination, and agility; helping to lower your risk of falls and injury, and should be added when ready.

Upper body progressions:
Assuming you are not reliant on an aid to assist with balance, practice by moving arms in a controlled and symmetrical way (arms opening and closing or raising and lowering). Progress to moving arms in a controlled asymmetrical pattern – one arm at a time. Other progressions include adding trunk rotations. Again, only progress if you feel safe doing so. As you progress, make sure there is support near you.

Visual progressions:
Progress to slowly dimming the lights or by wearing sunglasses. Dimming the lights or wearing sunglasses limits the visual information we process, making it harder to keep our balance. Only with the aid of another person should you consider closing your eyes. THIS IS NOT A SAFE PLACE TO START, but a future goal to work towards. By taking away all your visual senses, it can cause falls. Always start in a wide stance and progress when you feel ready and safe.

As always, practice and progress safely.

How does this help you Be Better?

Balance training should be integrated in your daily activities because it strengthens the core stabilizer muscles, builds body awareness, aids in daily movement, and allows us to live more independently.

Balance training improves muscle strength in the core which aids in keeping us upright. With improved muscle strength it is easier to keep balanced and recover from potential falls.

Balancing builds both coordination and body awareness by encouraging focus and concentration. Consistent balance training can help you learn about your body's abilities and capabilities and can help you improve them.

This is important because balance is essential for all movement tasks. Whenever we shift weight, we must maintain our balance. We shift weight while walking, squatting, standing, changing direction, jumping, pushing, and pulling. Practicing balance leads to being able to shift weight during our day-to-day tasks more easily and confidently. Allowing more independence.

I was out walking with my aunt, the same one mentioned in the Ankle Alphabet homework, on a snowy day. My aunt is in her early 60s and will not let that stop her from doing anything. During our walk, she stepped on a patch of ice. A fall on icy concrete would be devastating to anyone, let alone a 60-year-old woman.

However, in that instance, multiple things happened at once. I watched my aunt's core engage which helped her to maintain balance. She instinctively lowered to a squat. I saw her arms work to balance her in the microsecond it took her proprioceptors to register the slippery patch. I reached out to her, as she grabbed my arm. My aunt has taken DECADES of yoga, Pilates, and other balance training exercises. Though I was glad I was there to "help," all that previous training is what really helped her maintain her balance.

The good news is it is never too late to start practicing balance training. These skills can be built and improved. Only you can decide where you start this chapter. Again, remember to be safe in your practice.

Is your area safe and free of obstacles? Do you have a chair or something to hold onto, just in case? Are you ready to safely practice your balance? Then, get started. Stand nice and tall, engage your core, and start where you feel safe.

8

Cat Cow / Bird Dog

Your homework everyday this week is to practice both Cat Cow and Bird Dog every day this week for at least one minute each.

Considerations: If you have wrist, shoulder, knee injury, do this seated. If you have neck pain, keep your neck neutral. If you are pregnant or have any other concerns, look up safe ways to practice within your ability. As always, work within your range of motion. If you experience any pain, consult your primary care physician or physical therapist.

How to do your homework: Both the Cat Cow posture and the Bird Dog exercise can be done standing, seated, or in the tabletop position.

CAT COW

Seated - Sit in good posture placing hands on the thigh. Deep breath in, lift your chin and gaze up, slight arch to the back while keeping the shoulders down and back, pushing the hips back. Slow exhale, chin comes forward toward the chest, bending the back while tucking in the hips. Deep breath in, arching the back, deep breath out, rounding the back.

Standing - Stand in good posture with feet hip distance apart. Place hands on thighs to brace yourself. Come into a shallow squat by bending the knees and pushing your hips back, making sure to keep your back straight. Deep breath in, lift your chin up, arch your back, and push your hips back. Slow breath out, tucking your chin and hips towards each other while rounding your back, making sure to engage your core. Deep breath in, arching the back, deep breath out rounding the back.

Floor - If you have sensitive knees, place a folded towel or blanket under your knees. We are going to get into a tabletop position. Knees go under the hips, hands under shoulders. Your hips and shoulders should be neutral and flat. Deep breath in, engage the core by trying to bring your belly button to your spine. Slow exhale, tuck your chin towards your hips, rounding your back. Deep breath in, lift your chin up, arching the back while bringing the core down, and push the hips back. Exhale, tucking the chin to the hips, engaging the core, and rounding the back.

Regardless of which position you chose, try to do this stretch for at least a minute. Make sure to go slowly and with control.

BIRD/DOG

Seated (great for people with mobility issues) - Sitting in good posture with the core engaged. Deep breath in, lifting the left knee as high as comfortable and the right arm up. On your exhale lower your arm and leg. Inhale lifting the other side. Returning it on your exhale.

Standing - Standing in good posture. Deep breath in, lifting the right knee and left arm. Make sure to engage the core. Your hips and shoulders should stay neutral. Try to lift your knee so your thigh is parallel with the floor. Exhale, lower both arm and knee. Deep breath in, lift the left knee and right arm. Exhale, lowering both. When you feel confident, you can slowly extend the time your leg is lifted. If needed, use a chair to help balance.

Floor - If you have sensitive knees, place a folded towel under them. Get into the tabletop position (hands under shoulders, shoulders down and back, back flat, and knees under hips). Making sure to engage the core and keep the back straight. When you inhale, slowly extend and lift your right leg and left arm. While lifting, it is important to make sure that you do not rotate the hips or the shoulders. Imagine a cup of water on your back that you do not want to spill on yourself. Then on your exhale, lower your arm and leg.

On your next inhale, lift the other side. On your exhale, return them.

Regardless of position, make sure the core is engaged. From here, challenge yourself to hold each lift for two breaths, then four. Over time, see if you can build up your core strength to hold for eight breaths. As always, start and progress slowly and only if you feel confident and safe doing so. If at any time you lose form, rest, reset, and restart when you are ready.

How does this help you Be Better?

The Cat Cow posture strengthens the core, aids digestion, and reduces stress. While the benefits of the Bird Dog exercise include building core stability, improving posture, and aiding coordination.

The Cat Cow posture increases the flexibility in the hips, spine, neck, and shoulders while increasing strength in the erector spinae (muscles that run parallel to the spine) and abdominal muscles. This not only strengthens the core but adds flexibility, which allows for easier daily movement, better posture, and a decrease in back and neck pain.

The rocking motion of the Cat Cow pose both compresses and releases the digestive organs which encourages movement of waste. The rocking movement increases circulation to the midsection, helping supply oxygen to the digestive organs to aid digestion.

The slow, steady breathing combined with the movement of the back allows for better function of the diaphragm and lungs. With better lung function, more oxygen goes to the brain, which decreases stress. Second, stretching and deep breathing releases endorphins which are the "feel good hormones," elevating a person's mood and mental well-being.

The Bird Dog exercise strengthens the muscles of the back, like the erector spinae. The back muscles maintain and keep our core strong and stable. You cannot have a strong core if your back is weak. Strengthening the core and back may reduce back pain by relieving pressure and tension on the lower back and improving posture.

The challenge and mindfulness required to complete the Bird Dog exercise builds self-awareness and coordination. The coordination required, paired with the core stability needed for the asymmetrical movement, increases balance as well.

The Cat Cow and Bird Dog exercises are essential to not only keeping your back flexible but also strong. The simple movements, even for just a minute or two each day, will bring you relief. I had a client come to me after class thanking me for introducing this homework as it helped her with lower back pain.

That said, what are we waiting for? Get into the proper position and posture, engaging the core. Try to do a minute of each exercise. Making sure to use slow, deep breaths.

PS Consider doing Cat Cow right before bed as it will put you in a calm, meditative, and relaxed mood right before bed.

9

Practice Big Steps

> *Your homework everyday this week is to march in place, bringing your knees as high as you can. Your goal is lifting your leg, so your thigh is parallel with the floor.*

Considerations: If you have balance, gait, or mobility issues, then I recommend starting in a shallow water pool (bust to armpit level water) and then progressing to land. Again, make sure to start small and build your skills before progressing.

If you are starting on land, consider practicing in front of a mirror or next to a table or wall to assist with balance. Also, make sure the area in which you are practicing is free from obstacles or hazards. Most importantly, do not progress until you feel safe to do so. You decide what feels good for you and what works well for you.

How to do your homework: Stand with your feet hip distance apart and in good posture, making sure to engage your core. Your arms should be at your side, without moving your upper body, lift your knee as high as you can, gently put it down, and switch sides. Your goal is to bring your thigh parallel to the floor, however, you DO NOT need to start there. If needed, use a brace or something to hold onto.

Start with high knees in place, for a minute or two. It is important that the first few times you do this, you go slow. Focus on your range of motion, build self-awareness and coordination, engage your core, and maintain your balance. The goal is to master control of movement before adding speed or range of motion. Make sure to engage the core and not to arch or bend the back as that can cause low back pain.

After you can safely do the basics, you can choose to progress to a faster pace, increasing your range of motion, marching forward, side to side, and even backwards (please do so facing a mirror for your safety).

If you feel comfortable and want more of a cardiovascular challenge, you can add arm movements. If you would like to incorporate resistance training, you can add hand weights. If you want to work on your agility training, take three steps to each side. If you want to practice your balance, you can hold the high knee.

As always, add progressions slowly and only if you feel comfortable and confident. If you lose form at any time, it is important to stop, reset, and restart.

How does this help you Be Better?

Marching in place with high knees builds muscle strength and endurance, promotes heart health, and increases balance and coordination.

Marching in place activates the muscles of the quadriceps, hamstrings, glutes, and core improving their muscle strength and endurance. Specifically, it strengthens the muscles that surround the knee. This has been shown to help alleviate pain for those with osteoarthritis of the knee. People who incorporate marching in place to their exercise routine prior to knee replacement surgery tend to have better post-surgery outcomes.

Marching in place, in good form, is a great way to get the heart pumping. Marching and high knees utilize more oxygen, which requires the heart to pump more efficiently. This builds cardiac endurance. The increase of heart rate increases the caloric expenditure, which can aid in weight loss and maintenance.

By forcing the body to maintain balance through exaggerated movements, marching in place improves balance and coordination. This may help prevent falls. Practicing "big steps," or high knees can help people avoid trip hazards like curbs, floor transitions, rugs, stairs, and tubs.

The purpose of this homework, like many in this section, is fall prevention. The goal with this lesson is to teach us how to safely navigate the potential fall hazards we may face. Looking through your home, you can find a few things you have to step over or around. Do you have transitional floor strips, floor rugs, frayed carpet, cords on the floor, stairs, a pet, or a shower/bath combo? These are common trip hazards that become harder to step over as you age.

Not only is it important to recognize the fall hazards around, but it is also imperative to be able to navigate the obstacles safely and successfully. By practicing big steps, you are teaching your body to be better able to overcome those trip hazards. It is my belief that building this cognition and muscle memory can help you avoid falls in the future.

So, look around you, are you in a safe place with no obstacles or fall hazards around? Do you have a way to look at your form? If the answer to both of those questions is yes, then it is safe to get into good posture and practice high knees. If you are fearful of falling, please do this with something to hold on to. As always, if you feel unstable or lose form, stop, reset, and restart. Start small and build up your skills slowly and safely.

10

Keep On Stepping

> *Your homework everyday this week is to walk. That's it, just keep on walking.*

How to do your homework: If you can add a walk around the block, park a few spaces away or a block down, take a walk on your break, walk extra aisles at the store (without adding anything to the cart). Whatever your choices are, walk. Get your steps.

While walking, remember to maintain a good posture. Shoulders should be down and back, and your core should be engaged. Walking in poor posture not only affects your breath control but also your neck and back.

Though people do not actively think about how they step, it is important for your ankle, hip and back health to step properly. To take a proper step, you want to land first on your heel, articulate the foot down to the ball of the foot, and then to the toe, pushing off the next step with your toe. Lifting in the same way, heel first, ball, then toe.

Sometimes people walk on the balls of their feet. This forces the muscles of the ankle, calf, and hips to work harder. It also does not allow for full range of motion in the muscles, tendons, and ligaments of the ankle, knee, and hip.

Sometimes people walk using a passive step. This occurs when the foot lands as a whole unit with no articulation or bend. When we take a passive step then it puts extra pressure on your feet, ankles, knees, hips, rear end, and lower back causing pain. This happens because the feet no longer absorbing the shock of movement, dispersing weight properly, and inefficiently propelling us forward.

Sometimes people do not wear the correct footwear while walking, either the shoes are the wrong size, or have the wrong traction for the exercise. These things can increase your risk of fall and injury as well as impact the quality of your walk.

How does this help you Be Better?

Walking regularly can improve many aspects of health. Walking is a gentle exercise that strengthens the body, decreases the risk of heart disease, and aids with weight goals. Moreover, it contributes to better mood, improved balance, and higher quality of independence.

Walking utilizes the muscles of the legs, glutes, back and core. Building core strength helps the back and core to maintain our center of gravity to stabilize us, improving balance. By continuing to take our steps every day, we improve cardiac output and efficiency. This helps in decreasing the risk of cardiovascular disease, stroke, and high blood pressure. Moreover, it can add to a calorie deficit to help one attain weight or fitness goals.

Walking in nature increases the production of neurotransmitters such as serotonin, dopamine, and endorphins. These neurotransmitters help decrease the feelings of stress and anxiety, while boosting mood, and helping you have a better night's rest. The ability to walk confidently is a main contributor to quality of life, independence, and well-being as we age. Walking allows us to maintain our independence for longer.

Unfortunately, many people keep a sedentary lifestyle, and if you are one of them, let me applaud you for taking initiatives to improve your life.

You may have heard that you need to walk roughly 10,000 steps a day for a healthy lifestyle. And while that is true, benefits are shown in people who consistently walk 8,000 steps a day.

To know where you are at, we need to know what you are currently doing. A pedometer is the best tool to do this. If you do not have one, consider purchasing one. There are many different options at different price points for your needs. Most smart phones also have a built in pedometer function, however, they are less reliable than wearable alternatives.

When you know your average steps per day, your homework is to add 100 to 200 steps a day to your step count for four or five days. Then maintain for three to four days. Continue this process until you reach 8,000 steps per day.

It is important to slowly add exercise, especially if you are new to fitness. Walking too much before you are ready can lead to pain and injury, especially in the hip flexors. So, add slowly. An extra 200 steps a day is about fifteen extra steps per hour you are awake.

So, are you ready to add your extra steps? Put the book down, stand tall, and enjoy a quick walk.

11

Tongue Training

> *Your homework everyday this week is to try two or three of these myofunctional (tongue) therapy exercises each day.*

Considerations: For your safety, please make sure your mouth is empty and void for these tongue stretches. You will be working your tongue in ways it is not used to, that said, go slow, add repetitions, and hold time slowly. As for every body part, stretching should not cause pain. If this causes pain, minimize the stretch. Suggested repetitions and hold times are averages from guides of speech pathologists and oropharyngeal professionals. Below are tongue exercises and how to do them.

How to do your homework: Pick two or three of the listed tongue exercises to complete every day in front of a mirror.

Tongue Posture Exercise - Bringing the top of your tongue to the roof of your mouth sealing it there then dropping your jaw to create as much space as possible. Hold the stretch for 3 breaths. Repeat 5 to 8 times.

Tongue extension and retraction - Stick out your tongue as far as you can, hold for three breaths, then pull your tongue in as far as you can and hold for three breaths. Repeat 5 times.

Tongue side to side - Stick your tongue out as far as you can, bring your tongue as far to the right as possible then slowly back to center, and then as far to the left as possible. Repeat 5 to 8 times.

Pushing on the molars - With the tip of your tongue, press as hard as you can on each of your four molars for 3 breaths. Repeat 3 to 5 times.

Brushing teeth with tongue - Using your tongue as a toothbrush to clean the front and back of all your teeth keeping your jaw as still as possible.

Tongue Clicks - Click your tongue for 30 seconds.

How does this help you Be Better?
These exercises strengthen the muscles of the tongue and mouth. Strengthening these muscles improves speech

annunciation and pronunciation, aids in the ability to swallow and breathe, and helps maintain our ability to smile. Tongue exercises improve the posture and positioning of the jaw and tongue, building strength and awareness of the muscles around the mouth.

The tongue is composed of two sections, the front, and the back. The front section of the tongue is used for things like speech, chewing, and moving food so it can be swallowed. This uses quick bursts of energy to do its actions and then it gets rest. The type of muscle fiber found on the front section of the tongue is called fast twitch muscle fibers.

Meanwhile, the back section of the tongue is used to maintain our airways and to root the tongue into the mouth. These actions are constant and require muscle endurance. The back of your tongue uses slow twitch muscle fibers, which provide sustained activity. These muscle fibers do very different things, like your tongue.

As we age, our muscle mass and muscle tone decrease. Unfortunately, our tongues are no different. Muscle strength, mass, and tone in our tongues decrease too. If tongue muscle strength weakens, it could lead to slurred speech, quieter speech volume, problems chewing and swallowing food, and not being able to emote. Most importantly, tongue weakness can lead to problems maintaining the airway, difficulty breathing, and sleep apnea. So, it is important to challenge and move our tongue.

What are you waiting for? Pick two or three of the listed exercises, sit in front of the mirror, and get started!

Part Two

FOR THE BELLY

"Your diet is a bank account. Good food choices are good investments."
– Bethany Frankel

"Exercise is king. Nutrition is queen. Put them together and you've got a kingdom."
– Jack LaLanne

"Eating healthy food fills your body with energy and nutrients. Imagine your cells smiling back at you and saying: 'Thank you!'"
– Karen Salmansohn

12

Food Log

> *Your homework everyday this week is to log all your meals for the week.*

Considerations: Our goal for this chapter is to establish better eating habits and the advice given is for the general population. If you suffer from an eating disorder, be mindful that this chapter may impact you. If needed, please seek professional guidance to assist you.

How to do your homework: Your homework this week is to log the meals you consume. You can write down your log, use a food journal app, or take a picture with your phone. Things to note are what is being eaten, when you eat, and why you are eating.

Considering everyone is different, each person is going to do this differently. Whichever option suits you best, is the one you should do.

How does this help you Be Better?

People eat subconsciously. Without even realizing it, we pass by and peek into the fridge or pantry. Sometimes we eat out of hunger, or thirst, boredom, or celebration. The goal of this chapter is to learn the behaviors around why we eat, so we can implement better habits if needed.

There is no way to exercise off a bad diet. It is much easier to change your eating habits than it is to work off excess calories that are consumed. The first way to recognize issues with our diet is to log it and hold ourselves accountable to our diets.

Multiple studies have found that people who utilize food logs lost more weight than the participants that did not. The frequency in which they logged had a direct correlation with how much they lost. In one study, participants were grouped into "rare," "consistent," and "inconsistent" food loggers. Throughout the yearlong study, only the "consistent" group showed consistent weight loss.

When clients come to me asking how best they can tone up or slim down, my first question is to ask about their diet. As someone who has tried most diets, I used to feel discouraged whenever I would hear that word. After self-reflection and work, I came to change my definition of diet.

Diet, to me, is what a person eats in a day. It does not matter what is eaten, everything eaten is part of a person's diet. That said, to understand how our diet affects our body, we must know what our diet consists of.

Due to food additives, food scientists, ease, and constant advertisements, food has become increasingly addictive. This makes it harder to stop eating, portion control, or eat healthier options. People often consume food without realizing it. You may even be reading this while enjoying a snack.

To recognize what we are eating, we need to log and keep track of our food intake. Important things to consider logging food are: what, when, and why.

What are you eating? What is in the food? What items can be replaced with healthier options? What are the portion sizes being consumed? When are you eating? Is there a tendency to eat extra at night? When do you normally eat your first meal? Why? Why are you eating right now? Are you hungry, sad, bored, celebrating an achievement?

Whatever you consume, write it down and study it once a week. If logging food is difficult for you, there are many apps that will allow you to take a picture of your plate and allow you to note your why.

In order to change and affect our habits, we need to be fully aware of them. That said, the following few pages are a quick food log for he week for you to start. So, let's get logging!

DAY 1
Breakfast
Meal _____
Time_____ Why_____

Lunch
Meal _____
Time_____ Why_____

Dinner
Meal _____
Time_____ Why_____

Snack 1
Meal _____
Time_____ Why_____

Snack 2
Meal _____
Time_____ Why_____

Snack 3
Meal _____
Time_____ Why_____

DAY 2
Breakfast
Meal _____
Time_____ Why_____

Lunch
Meal _____
Time_____ Why_____

Dinner
Meal _____
Time_____ Why_____

Snack 1
Meal _____
Time_____ Why_____

Snack 2
Meal _____
Time_____ Why_____

Snack 3
Meal _____
Time_____ Why_____

DAY 3

Breakfast
Meal _____
Time_____ Why_____

Lunch
Meal _____
Time_____ Why_____

Dinner
Meal _____
Time_____ Why_____

Snack 1
Meal _____
Time_____ Why_____

Snack 2
Meal _____
Time_____ Why_____

Snack 3
Meal _____
Time_____ Why_____

DAY 4

Breakfast
Meal _____
Time_____ Why_____

Lunch
Meal _____
Time_____ Why_____

Dinner
Meal _____
Time_____ Why_____

Snack 1
Meal _____
Time_____ Why_____

Snack 2
Meal _____
Time_____ Why_____

Snack 3
Meal _____
Time_____ Why_____

DAY 5
Breakfast
Meal _____
Time_____ Why_____

Lunch
Meal _____
Time_____ Why_____

Dinner
Meal _____
Time_____ Why_____

Snack 1
Meal _____
Time_____ Why_____

Snack 2
Meal _____
Time_____ Why_____

Snack 3
Meal _____
Time_____ Why_____

DAY 6

Breakfast
Meal _____
Time_____ Why_____

Lunch
Meal _____
Time_____ Why_____

Dinner
Meal _____
Time_____ Why_____

Snack 1
Meal _____
Time_____ Why_____

Snack 2
Meal _____
Time_____ Why_____

Snack 3
Meal _____
Time_____ Why_____

DAY 7

Breakfast
Meal _____
Time_____ Why_____

Lunch
Meal _____
Time_____ Why_____

Dinner
Meal _____
Time_____ Why_____

Snack 1
Meal _____
Time_____ Why_____

Snack 2
Meal _____
Time_____ Why_____

Snack 3
Meal _____
Time_____ Why_____

13

Buy the Rainbow, Eat the Rainbow

> *Your homework for this week is to buy fruits and vegetables (including legumes) from every color of the rainbow. Your second piece of homework is to eat them all before they go bad.*

How to do your homework: The next time you go grocery shopping, pick at least one fruit or vegetable from each color of the rainbow. If you want, try out a new recipe or enjoy an old recipe. It is up to you, but make sure you eat your delicious fruits and vegetables.

Fruit and vegetables ideas per color.

Red fruits: grapes, apples, cherries, watermelon, strawberries, and raspberries. Red vegetables: bell peppers, red cabbage, beets, radishes, tomatoes, kidney beans, and chard.

Orange fruits: oranges, tangerines, cantaloupes, mangoes, and peaches. Orange vegetables: acorn and butternut squash, carrots, bell peppers, and sweet potatoes.

Yellow fruits: pineapple, lemon, star fruit, papaya, and quince. Yellow vegetables: summer squash, corn, and bell peppers.

Green fruits: green apples, green grapes, honeydew melon, and kiwi. Green vegetables: Brussel sprouts, broccoli, avocado, asparagus, green beans, snap peas, cucumbers, and celery.

Blue and purple fruits: blueberries, blackberries, plums, prunes, acai, and dates. Blue and purple vegetables: eggplant, purple carrots, purple yams, and taro.

White fruits: coconut, bananas, dragon fruit, and lychee. White vegetables: cauliflower, mushrooms, potatoes, turnips, and parsnips.

How does this help you Be Better?

The variety of colors found in fruits and vegetables occur because there are different plant pigmentations that give each fruit and vegetable their color. These colors each have different chemical compounds resulting in different health benefits.

Red fruits and vegetables contain plant pigments called anthocyanins and lycopene. They are both antioxidants with anti-inflammatory properties. They protect the skin from UV induced damage and may help prevent sunburn. Both have properties to help with cancer preventions. Lycopene also helps with eye health.

Orange and yellow fruits and vegetables contain carotenoids. Carotenoids promote eye health, offer skin protection, contain anti-inflammatory properties, potential cancer prevention (breast, prostate, colon, skin, and lung cancer), lower bad cholesterol, improve blood vessel function, and protect your nervous system.

Green fruits and vegetables contain lutein and folate. Lutein is a type of carotenoid and is known to promote eye health, help lower the risk of heart disease and may reduce the risk of cognitive decline. Leafy green vegetables contain folate, which is a B vitamin that promotes healthy cell growth and blood cell production. Vitamin B is extremely important in promoting healthy pregnancies.

Anthocyanins occur in blue, purple and, red fruits and vegetables. Anthocyanins have properties like being an antioxidant, antimicrobial, and anti-inflammatory, as well as helping prevent certain cancers. And they help keep the heart and brain healthy.

White vegetables contain anthoxanthins which may help maintain a strong immune system, lower blood pressure, bad cholesterol, and reduce risk of heart disease and cancer.

A variety of fruits and vegetables are important to maintaining many facets of your health. Your homework this week is to buy at least ONE fruit and/or vegetable of each color group. Switch out a snack for fruits or vegetables. Add fruit to breakfast, or veggies to your lunch or dinner.

Part two of the homework is to eat all the fruits and vegetables before it goes bad. You get bonus points for trying a new recipe.

So, which fruits and vegetables are you going to get this week?

RED:
FRUITS _____
VEGETABLES _____

ORANGE:
FRUITS _____
VEGETABLES _____

YELLOW:
FRUITS _____
VEGETABLES _____

GREEN:
FRUITS _____
VEGETABLES _____

BLUE/PURPLE:
FRUITS _____
VEGETABLES _____

WHITE:
FRUITS _____
VEGETABLES _____

14

Eat This First

> *Your homework everyday this week is to add at least one serving of either fruit or vegetables to every meal. Then, eat that first.*

How to do your homework: Eat your fruit and vegetables. How you do that is up to you. You can steam them, bake them, boil and mash them. You can slice them, dice them, chop them, or grate them. You can stew them or eat them raw. But you must eat them. When preparing your fruits and vegetables, be mindful of dressings and toppings.

How does this help you Be Better?

As stated in the previous chapters, fruits and vegetables are great for your body's processes. The vitamins and minerals provided by a diet rich in fruits and vegetables allow the body to function as efficiently and effectively as possible.

Fruits and vegetables contain dietary fiber which is essential for our digestive tract. It helps move waste along and prevent constipation. In cases of chronic constipation, foods like apples, pears, broccoli, and sweet potatoes can help. Moreover, a diet high in fiber can reduce risks of hemorrhoids, colon disease, and colorectal cancer.

It is important to eat fruits and vegetables first. Eating fruits and vegetables first encourages the body to fill up on nutrient and mineral rich foods. These foods assist in feeling full because they are high in fiber and water, which also contributes to overall hydration.

Dietary fiber also lowers bad cholesterol and reduces the risk of heart disease, stroke, diabetes, and some types of cancer. Further, a diet high in vegetables has a positive effect on blood sugar. Fruit, in moderation and as an alternative to high sugar snacks, has a similar effect on blood sugar. However, some fruits and vegetables are better for your blood sugar than others.

Foods can be classified by the glycemic index. This index measures how quickly food is digested and processed for energy. Foods high on the glycemic index are quickly digested and processed, releasing a short burst of energy and spiking blood sugar. To compensate for blood sugar increase, the pancreas releases insulin. This can cause the blood sugar to drop, which activates the pancreas to release the hormone glucagon to help raise and stabilize the blood sugar. These fluctuations can damage the pancreas, making it less functional, and leading to diabetes. Processed foods tend to be high on the glycemic index.

Many fruits and vegetables have a low glycemic index. Foods low on the glycemic index are slowly digested and processed into energy. The energy provided is longer lasting. Foods low on the glycemic index are slow to elevate the blood sugar leading to less insulin and glucagon being released by the pancreas

Again, be considerate of the toppings that go on your fruits and vegetables. By adding a tablespoon or two of our favorite dressing, sauce, butter, or cheese we also add extra calories, fats, and sodium. Be cognizant of how you prepare your food.

Regardless of how they are prepared, eat your fruit and vegetable portion first. At least one serving per meal. Every meal this week.

15

Half a Plateful of Fruits and Veggies

> *Your homework every meal this week is to fill at least half your plate with fruits, vegetables, or both.*

How to do your homework: When serving yourself your meals this week, be mindful of what your meal comprised of. One half of each meal should be fruits and vegetables, a quarter protein, and the last quarter with carbohydrates or grains.

I know how hard it is to fill half the plate with fruits and vegetables. If that is hard for you too, start with a third of the plate and gradually progress to half the plate being fruits and vegetables. The important thing is to continue to build habits of healthy eating, including a variety of produce.

You get bonus points: for trying a new recipe with at least two fruits or veggies.

How does this help you Be Better?

As stated in the previous chapters, fruits and vegetables provide so many benefits.

The vitamins and minerals provided by fruits and vegetables help increase bone density and mass, lowering the risk of osteoporosis. The fiber in fruits and vegetables helps the intestines to be more efficient at absorbing amino acids, therefore aiding muscle growth.

Fruits and vegetables lower bad cholesterol and has been associated with lowering the risk of cardiovascular disease. Eating fruits and vegetables help prevent cognitive decline, making them brain healthy too.

However, fruits and vegetables cannot be the only aspect of our diet. We also need a healthy balance of proteins and carbohydrates.

Proteins play a significant role in muscle repair and growth. The amino acids provided in proteins are synthesized to repair and grow muscles. Protein also has a role in bone formation and density. Adequate protein allows for production of hormones that encourage calcium absorption and bone growth and repair.

Protein affects your metabolism through muscle mass, hormone manipulation, and increasing body temperature. Protein encourages muscle gain which changes the body composition. Muscle mass helps speed up the metabolism. Protein reduces the hormone Ghrelin which is known as the "hunger" hormone. Ghrelin slows the metabolism and reduces the ability to metabolize and burn fat. Moreover, protein takes more energy to digest. This raises the core temperature and increases metabolic function.

Carbohydrates can be either simple or complex. Simple carbohydrates provide a quick burst of energy. The simple structure allows for fast metabolism. Often, processed foods contain simple carbohydrates. The more processed the food is, the easier it is to metabolize and the faster it is to burn our energy out. This can lead to instability of energy levels. It can also lead to inconsistent blood sugar levels, which can overexert the pancreas leading to diabetes.

Complex carbohydrates take more effort to break down and get the energy from. This leads to slower and more consistent energy absorption and blood sugar levels. Complex carbohydrates are found in brown rice, quinoa, couscous, barley, and whole grain oats. However, one of the best sources of complex carbohydrates are vegetables, legumes and fruits, like: chickpeas, lentils, peas, sweet potatoes, corn, berries, apples, and bananas.

I know, I keep discussing the benefits of fruits and vegetables. I also know they are not always the most appetizing option. However, they are the healthiest options for our body. If we want to live as long and healthy as possible, then we need to take a good look at what we eat.

I get those thoughts, chips or carrots? I know which one I want, but I also know which one my body needs. I know that the convenience of these fast-food options have led many, including myself, to unhealthy lifestyles. I know that my body does not feel as good when I eat processed foods. I know how much better I feel when I make healthier choices.

Is it easy? No. Does it get easier with time and practice? Yes. Is it easier when we have more healthy options available? Yes.

So, on your next meal, think about what you are eating. Is at least half fruit or veggies? If not, go add some. Enjoy your meals this week! Again, bonus points for recipes with plenty of veggies.

16

Salad Plate

> *Your homework everyday this week is to use a salad plate for your each of your meals.*

In this chapter, we will be discussing general information on portions and servings. However, everybody and every body is different. If you have any questions, please contact a registered dietitian to assist you and your needs.

How to do your homework: Switch out the larger entree plate for the smaller salad plate.

How does this help you Be Better?

Changing out your entree plate is crucial in changing the way our brains process the amount of food we eat.

To understand why, we need to discuss two terms. The first term is "serving size," and the second term is "portion." Serving size is the amount of food listed on the food label.

The information provided on the food label shows the fat, calories, sodium, etc. in the product per that serving. The serving size is there to help consumers understand their food choices. For example, a serving size for a loaf of bread is one slice. The portion is how many servings are consumed. There may be more than one serving consumed in one portion. For example, eating two slices of bread when having a sandwich.

Adjusting the portions eaten can assist with weight loss and maintenance. A simple way to adjust our portions is to change our serving plate. This is important because it is hard to imagine the correct SERVING SIZE when we put our PORTION on a large plate. When there is a lot of room on the plate, the first impulse is to fill it. And when we put food on the plate, our next impulse is to try and eat it all.

Smaller portions are easier for the body to digest properly, reducing the risk of heartburn and acid reflux, and aids in the absorption of the nutrients needed for the body. On the other hand, larger portion sizes can lead to unstable blood sugar levels. Unstable blood sugar levels impact the pancreas, the organ which is responsible for blood sugar regulation.

Eating on a salad plate limits portion sizes. Look at the size difference between a salad plate and an entree plate. The salad plate is roughly eight inches in diameter, giving you roughly fifty square inches of plate to eat off. The entree plate is about ten inches, giving seventy-eight square inches for one plate. Think of how much extra food is added onto the entree plate.

By switching out one large plate for a smaller one, we can dramatically decrease the amount of food we are eating. If you are still hungry after five to ten minutes after eating (how long it takes for the stomach and brain to communicate how full you are), then give yourself permission to have more, but be careful of what and how much you are getting.

17

Drink Your Water

> *Your homework everyday this week is to drink more water. That's it.*

How to do your homework: Strive to drink at least eight glasses of water a day. If you are not currently drinking this much water, strive to add half a glass of water to your daily intake until you get to eight glasses of water a day. Be mindful not to overhydrate.

How does this help you Be Better?
Water keeps your body working effectively. It is essential for healthy circulation and thermoregulation, oral hygiene, and body waste removal. Extra benefit, it is good for the wallet, too.

Proper hydration helps thin out the blood, improving blood circulation. Better circulation means the heart is working more effectively and efficiently. Better blood circulation also helps to regulate body temperature.

When body temperature increases, the body perspires and the evaporation of the sweat cools the skin. When the body is cool, water in the body acts as a conductor of heat that helps to retain heat. Proper hydration is required for proper thermoregulation.

With proper brushing and flossing, staying hydrated aides in oral health and cavity prevention. Saliva is used to wash away debris, sugars, and plaque from our teeth. Adequate hydration allows the right amount of saliva to wash away the debris and prevent them from sticking to our teeth, helping prevent oral cavities. Saliva is made up of roughly 90% water. The rest is composed of different minerals like calcium, magnesium, and phosphates which strengthens the enamel of your teeth. Drinking water plays an essential role to preventing tooth decay.

Saliva also has enzymes that assist in chewing and breaking down our foods. After swallowing, food journeys to the stomach where hydration plays a role in producing the acid to further break down the food. When our food is next processed in the intestines, water helps absorb the water-soluble vitamins and minerals. Proper hydration also allows for softer bowel movements.

Without proper hydration, the kidneys cannot remove waste from the blood as efficiently. This can cause a lack of urine, kidney damage, chronic kidney disease, urinary tract infections, and kidney stones. Water helps remove the waste from the kidneys. If there is not enough water, then waste cannot be properly removed.

There are so many positives to drinking enough water. That said, you can drink too much water which can lead to overhydration or water intoxication. Overhydration can cause electrolyte imbalances in your body with symptoms ranging from nausea, vomiting, cramping, headaches, and lightheadedness.

According to the Mayo Clinic, the signs of dehydration include extreme thirst, infrequent urination, fatigue, confusion, dizziness, and dryness of your lips, mouth, and skin. The body can also confuse dehydration for hunger, so at times when we feel hungry, we are actually thirsty.

Your climate, medicine or medical conditions, and activity levels can all impact the amount of water need to be properly hydrated. You can tell how hydrated you are by your urine. If it's too pale or even clear, it means the waste has been diluted by too much water. If your urine is pale yellow, you are properly hydrated. If your urine is dark yellow, it means there is not enough water to dilute the waste properly. Generally, properly hydrated people urinate around six to eight times a day.

If water is not something you typically drink, start small. Consider how much water you typically drink in a day. If you find that most of your beverages are not water, slowly incorporate a glass of water before having your other drink of choice. If you are not getting the recommended amount of water right now, that's okay! Challenge yourself to add a half cup a day of water until you reach the recommended amount of eight glasses a day. Your body will be so thankful and appreciative.

So, grab your water, and cheers to another chapter completed!

Part Three

FOR THE SOUL

"Put your heart, mind, and soul into even your
smallest acts. This is the secret to success."
- Swami Sivananda

"How much good inside a day?
Depends on how you live them."
- Shel Silverstein

"It is so important to take time for yourself
and find clarity. The most important relationship
is the one you have with yourself."
- Diane Von Furstenberg

18
Three Kind Choices

> *Your homework everyday this week is to make three kind choices a day. One for a loved one, one for a stranger, and one for yourself.*

How to do your homework: Make a kind choice for a loved one. Whether it is checking in on a neighbor, reading to a child, doing the dishes, offering a hug or a shoulder to lean on, checking in on a friend, or making a favorite meal. Make a kind choice for someone important to you.

Make a kind choice for a stranger. It could be letting the person with one thing at the store go in front of you, helping someone get something, letting the person merge in front of you, donating to a charity, or making time to volunteer.

Make a kind choice for yourself. It could be taking time to stretch, read, exercise, meditate, or eat healthier. All of those are kind choices you can make for you and your body.

How does this help you Be Better?
KINDNESS MATTERS.

Other reasons to make kind choices include fostering better relationships, boosting your and others' moods, and helping keep the heart healthy.

Being kind to friends, family, coworkers, and strangers impacts your relationships with them for the better. Kind people are surrounded by more people, which can combat the feelings of loneliness and depression. More importantly, our actions ripple. Recent studies have found that when we are kind and compassionate to others, it makes them want to be kind to someone else. Moreover, when kindness is witnessed, the people who see it make kinder choices. In this way, you can spread kindness to multiple people in one action.

Being kind releases both serotonin and oxytocin. Serotonin is responsible for our overall feelings and wellbeing; and oxytocin, is known as the "love hormone," appears to be associated with love, trust, and bonding. Oxytocin also triggers a response that dilates blood vessels, decreasing blood pressure.

Being kind reduces stress and the hormone cortisol. Cortisol has many functions in our body, including stress response. When we are stressed the body releases cortisol.

Too much cortisol can lead to high blood pressure, weight gain, mood changes, and osteoporosis.

One time when this was a homework assignment, I was the recipient of a random act of kindness. During that week, I forgot to take my garbage bins out. I noticed as soon as I started driving my child to school, making a note to take them out when I got home. As soon as I parked my car, still in my pajamas and house slippers, I saw the garbage truck at my next-door neighbor's house. The garbage truck could have easily gone past me, but they waited an extra minute for me to make it down my driveway, with my garbage bins.

That simple act of kindness made my day. And while I was giving homework the rest of that week, I shared that story. That little action had an impact on me and my clients who heard about it that week. Actions of kindness do not have to be big, because little actions make a big difference. It can be as simple as waiting an extra minute, a word of encouragement, opening a door, or taking time to better yourself.

Spending time reading this chapter means you have made a kind choice for yourself, so you are one third through with your homework! Way to go! I am so proud of you.

19

Reach Out

> *Your homework everyday this week is to reach out to someone if they pop into your mind. Call, text, e-mail, facetime, – it does not matter. Just reach out and let them know.*

How to do your homework: As you go about your day and someone comes into your mind, reach out and let them know. Share how they impacted you for the better and made you into who you are today. Whether it be an inside joke, a good memory, a song, a recipe, whatever. If you think about them, let them know.

How does this help you Be Better?

Staying connected, especially as we get older and our lives change, is increasingly difficult. However, studies have shown the positive effects that reaching out has, including stress reduction, improved mental and emotional health, and maintained friendships.

Reaching out can impact not only your mental and emotional health, but theirs as well. It reduces stress and leads to a longer lifespan. People are social creatures and reaching out is a gentle way to remind people they matter and belong, reducing the feelings of isolation and loneliness. This feeling can bring them into a better mental space to make kinder, more empathetic choices throughout their day, affecting more people.

Conversations allow us to deepen the connections of the people in our lives and help build new ones. In the digital age, it is getting harder to maintain real life relationships. A simple call, text, or e-mail can bridge that gap. Andy Stanley, an American Pastor, stated, "Every conversation is a construction zone and we're either building or tearing down with our words." When you reach out, don't forget to "build" up.

I cannot stress the importance of reaching out and interacting with the people who surround you. Whether it be colleagues, friends, or family. Let people know they have impacted you for the better and have helped shape you into who you are now. Reiterating from the previous chapter, kindness is transferable. Meaning that one kind act brings about another. It ripples and affects farther than we know.

I remember teaching an Ai Chi class and a new member came. At the end I gave this homework. The following week, she stopped me and thanked me. She told me about how she reached out to her uncle; someone she had not connected much with after her mom passed. They shared a great conversation, told stories, and agreed to keep in touch better.

One simple call affected not only my client but also her uncle. It also impacted all the interactions they made throughout the day. And hearing her story impacted me.

Reach out and remind people important to you that they matter.

20

Meditate

> *Your homework everyday this week is to practice meditating for three to eight minutes each day.*

Before you start this homework, understand there are many types of meditation and some may work for you, and some may not. It is okay to practice and decide if what you are doing is working.

There are many tools like apps, videos, and books that offer guided meditation. These typically focus on mindfulness meditation, focused meditation, and visualizations. Other types include spiritual and movement meditation. Movement meditation offer movement and a mind body connection like QiGong, Yoga, Tai Chi, Ai Chi, or a walk in nature. Movement meditations encourage mental and physical balance.

How you chose to meditate is up to you. As always, mediation is a practice, and you should start small.

How to do your homework: First, let's sit down. The most important aspect to any meditative practice is breathing. To breathe properly, we need to do a posture check. Ears over shoulders, shoulders down and back, core engaged, hip under shoulders. Put one hand on your heart, and the other on your belly. Breathe in through your nose, breathe out through your mouth.

Breathe in a little bit slower now. Pause for a second, exhale slowly through your mouth. Breathe in just a little bit slower. Feel how your chest and stomach inflate and fill. Slowly breathe out. Deep, slow breath in, pause, and slow breath out. Continue the slow calming rhythm. Deep breath in, pause, slow breath out.

On your inhale, imagine breathing peace and love into your heart. On your exhale, imagine breathing out all the frustrations you may be holding on to. Deep breath in, breathing in the good. Focus on the good. Slow breath out, breathing out the bad. Deep breath in, feeling calmness and relaxation. Deep breath out. Deep breath in feeling peace.

Pause on thoughts of peace. Deep breath out. On your inhale, imagine your happy place, a place or a moment that fills your heart with joy. Slow breath out. Deep breath in, imagine your happy place, deep breath out. Breathe deeply for thirty breaths and imagine. Close your eyes.

Great Job! You just completed your mediation homework, and I am immensely proud of you! I would like you to reflect on how you feel right now. I have left you some space below to write down your thoughts and feelings.

_____
_____
_____
_____
_____
_____
_____
_____
_____
_____

How does this help you Be Better?

The benefits of meditation are as varied as the types and ways to meditate. Meditation gives people the opportunity to slow down and focus on the moment. Building concentration, focus, self-awareness, self-reflection, and mindfulness. It builds empathy and compassion and helps people become more present in their relationships.

Again, there are multiple ways to meditate. Above was a combination of both visualization and breath awareness. I suggest you try other mindfulness and guided meditation.

Meditation can be used before a difficult task to build self-confidence or as a way to calm and relax. For instance, before I debut new song to my dance class, I visualize it to commit it to memory and to build my confidence. However, my favorite meditation is the body scan, where you focus on the sensations of how the body feels. I like to do that before bed to calm my mind and help me get to sleep.

I suggest you try out different methods and find what works for you. Good news, you get to spend three to eight minutes each day this week to practice a new one, or to find a new favorite one.

I hope this week brings you confidence, peace, self-awareness, and relaxation.

21

Sunshine and Sunscreen

> *Your homework everyday this week is to put on some sunscreen and enjoy some time outside.*

How to do your homework: The homework this week is simple enough. Just put on your sunscreen and enjoy time outside. You can sit and read a book, you can take some extra steps and enjoy a walk, put on music and do a little dance, work in a garden, or take a moment to meditate and be thankful. There are plenty of things to do outside. Just make sure you put the devices down and the sunscreen on.

How does this help you Be Better?

Sunscreen is the best defense against sun damage that the sun can cause. Wearing sunscreen regularly protects the skin from UV rays which can cause skin cancer, wrinkles, and premature aging. UV rays are present regardless of the weather, so it is important to wear sunscreen even on cloudy days.

Sunscreen provides an extra layer of protection from the pollutants. This fights hyper-pigmentation of the skin, helping maintain an even skin tone. The hydration provided by sunscreen makes your skin less likely to have skin irritations. Added benefit, lotions and moisturizers now include sunscreen, so it is easy to find and use.

Spending time outside increases the synthesis of vitamin D. Vitamin D helps with calcium regulation, bone health, weight loss, cancer prevention, and immunity health. Though there are dietary sources and vitamins to help supplement, UVB rays from the sun help our body synthesize vitamin D so our body can properly absorb and utilize it.

There are differing opinions about the effectiveness of vitamin D synthesis while wearing sunscreen. Some specialists note that wearing sunscreen mildly inhibits the synthesis. However, most dermatologists agree that the benefit of skin protection outweighs this.

Being outdoors and in nature has been shown to help reduce depression, stress, and blood pressure. This contributes to better cardiovascular health. Typically, when we are outdoors, we are also doing physical activity such as walking, gardening, or biking which also benefits our heart health.

Natural light helps regulate and reset the circadian cycle. The circadian cycle is our internal clock and assists us in waking and sleeping by releasing hormones to wake us up and to help us relax for sleep. This reset of the circadian cycle can aid in a better night's sleep.

Regardless of the weather, you need sunscreen. Both UVA and UVB can damage your skin even on cloudy days. We cannot see these rays, but they still impact and can harm our body. Regardless of your race, you need to wear sunscreen. People of color can and do get skin cancer. Because it is less studied, it takes longer for people of color to get a diagnosis and treatment. This leads to worse outcomes.

If you are spending a long day in the sun, make sure to reapply your sunscreen regularly. Let's take a walk to your moisturizers and lotions. Do any of them provide sun protection? If so, put the book down so you can hydrate and protect your skin. If not, pick some up on your next trip to the store.

Now, for part two of the homework. How are you going to enjoy the outdoors today? A short walk, reading a book under a tree, a little bit of gardening or birdwatching? Regardless of how you choose to enjoy the outdoors this week, take a deep breath and enjoy your time.

22

Try Something New

> Your homework in this section is to try something new each day this week.

How to do your homework: Find a new recipe, game, or book. Explore a new restaurant, trail, or store. Try a new fitness class, podcast, or hobby. Practice a new language, skill, or instrument. It does not matter, just try something new.

How does this help you Be Better?

Trying new things is so good for our mental and emotional wellbeing. Not only does trying something new help alleviate boredom, but it also leads to improved confidence, new skills, and brain stimulation.

Trying new skills, even when we are not successful, is a confidence booster. By trying something new, we prove to ourselves that we can do it, even if we previously thought we would not be able. We gain a new skillset and confidence in that skill. By learning a new skill, we gain knowledge.

This stimulates different sections of the brain. For those sections to communicate with each other, they need to send communications or synapses. By learning new things, our brain builds more connections to communicate, improving brain health and longevity. Moreover, by exposing ourselves to new things, it leads to more innovative thinking which can spark and stimulate creativity in your way of thought.

Trying new things is a great way to invest your time. It allows you to learn more about yourself and your interests. It is important to celebrate any and all successes and grant yourself time to improve new skills. No one is asking for perfection, just a willingness to try a new thing. It may go well, or it may fail miserably. Either way, it's okay.

I remember walking past a sushi rolling kit in the store with my child who loves sushi. They wanted it, so we got one. I bought the ingredients to try sushi at home. It was not a disaster, but it was not a total success either. I could not get the rice right. The fish would not cut properly. I had too many vegetable options. I decided to wing it and hope for the best. Anyway, we enjoyed the meal, with lots of laughs. The next time I made sushi, I knew how to better prepare everything. I knew how to make an assembly line. By the third attempt, I realized that less ingredients had better outcomes. By the fourth or fifth sushi making experience, I was making it for friends and family. It was not perfect, but it was amazing. And now my child and I enjoy making sushi together.

The reason this book has come about was because when I gave this to my class as their homework, they challenged me to write a book as my try something new. To those who were in that class, thank you for inspiring me to do this. It has boosted my confidence, stimulated my creativity, and helped me avoid countless hours of boredom (though they are now filled with editing)!

I want you to feel this confidence, this creativity, this newfound joy of discovering new interests, and that is why Trying Something New is your homework this week.

Now, let's talk about some ground rules.

1. YOU DON'T HAVE TO BE PERFECT. Rome was not built in a day, and it is silly to think anything new you try will be perfect. No one is expecting perfection, just courage and bravery to try something new.

2. Laugh often. If you find a moment to laugh, do it. If everything is going wrong, laugh about it. If everything is going right, laugh about that too.

3. Start small and prepare. How do you climb a big mountain? One small step at a time. Likewise, you would not climb a big mountain without the proper equipment or knowledge. You would want all the knowledge you can get to avoid common mistakes. You need to prepare.

4. Give yourself grace and love. It takes so much courage to try something new. You got this.

So what fun things are you ready to explore? Go out and do it, I believe in you!

23

Read

> *Your homework everyday this week is to spend at least thirty minutes reading.*

How to do your homework: Listen to or read for thirty minutes a day. Spend at least fifteen minutes of that time learning about something to improve or expand your knowledge base. Try not to read on a screen as the blue light can affect your eyes and focus. Find something to read or listen to (yes, audiobooks count). It does not matter if it is something you have already read, a new magazine, or a news article. Just make sure you read.

Local libraries offer plenty of options, in both book and audiobook form, for whatever genre entices you. If you return borrowed items in a timely manner, then it is a free service. Though, sometimes you may be put on a waitlist.

If you are lucky enough to have one nearby, there are little neighborhood libraries which offer much more limited options. If libraries are not your thing, then there are many cafes in which you can sit down, enjoy a beverage, and read a book.

Whichever option works best for you, make sure you find a book that interests you. This is your time to relax and unwind. This homework pairs nicely with Put Down The Devices, Sunshine and Sunscreen, and Learning Something New.

How does this help you Be Better?

There are intrinsic effects of reading like growing your knowledge base, vocabulary, and creativity. Reading also promotes better sleep and lowers stress by providing an escape from the day to day.

There are extrinsic benefits like gaining different perspectives to grow our critical thinking skills, being better able to navigate day-to-day interactions, and improved communication skills.

Multiple studies have shown that regular reading can improve memory. The act of reading requires multiple parts of your brain to process and understand the words read. As previously stated, when multiple parts of the brain communicate, it helps build connections and brain longevity.

Reading is one of the most important things a person can do. It allows us to learn, to escape, to fantasize, and to self-reflect. It helps us be brave, learn compassion, and gain critical thinking skills. It gives us time to disassociate from the day to day and focus on what we want our minds to focus on.

I am proud of you for taking the time to read today and better yourself. Thank you for starting this week with this book. I wish you plenty of adventures, daring escapes, funny stories, some self-reflection, and time to relax this week with your homework.

Happy Reading!

24

Put Down the Screens

> *Your homework everyday this week is to carve out two hours without screen time, one of those hours should be right before you go to bed. You can listen to meditations, or gentle music, just do not look at screens or devices.*

How to do your homework: Do not look at your screen for two hours of your day. Again, you listen to an audiobook, podcast, or music. Just no looking at the screen. You can break this time up into two or three screen free periods, but at least one hour should be right before your bedtime.

This homework combines very well with much of the homework provided in this book. If you are going screen free earlier in the day, consider practicing either agility or balance training, or high knees. In the middle of the day, maybe get in some steps with a walk, try a new fitness or dance class, enjoy time outside, or go to the library.

For your screen free hour before bed, consider taking time to relax and heal your body. Stretching, and the cat cow posture rely on slowing your breath. This calms the body and helps bring the body to rest. If you want, you can read or meditate as both help relax you to a restful state. Think of this time as your time to recover, relax, and reset from the day.

How does this help you Be Better?

There are many negative effects that screen usage has on our body and minds.

Too much screen time can lead to obesity. Sitting in front of screens leads to inactivity. When we are inactive, our body does not work off the calories that we consume. Moreover, people eat regularly in front of screens.

Typically, it is extremely difficult to stay in good posture while using screens. This poor posture can lead to neck and back pain as discussed in Posture Checks. Which reminds me, are you in good posture right now? Have you done a posture check recently? Let's do one right now. Ears above shoulders, shoulders down and back, lengthening the spine. Ask yourself, "Does my neck feel stiff?" Answer, "Yes," "I don't know," "No," and "Whoooohoooo."

The blue light that emits from most screens can cause temporary eye strain. Often when staring at devices, the blinking rate decreases, the eyes become dry, and there is eye strain from focusing intently on an object close to the eyes.

Further, the constant exposure of blue light emitted from the screens may cause retinal cell damage and macular degeneration.

The blue light tricks our body into thinking it is still daytime. This hinders the circadian cycle making it harder for our brains to turn off to go to bed. Studies show that people who do not use screens before bed tend to sleep better and wake up more refreshed.

Positives that occur when we put down and stop looking at the screens are, improved neck, spine, and core health. Free time to be creative, take better care of yourself, and do other things. Most importantly, it allows you to be more present in the real-life interactions that occur around you.

I know how hard it is to be without my phone, or to have no electronics going. But I also know, my interactions with my family are better for it. I know how much easier it is to fall asleep when I have not been watching tv for the hour before bed. I know how much better my body feels when I stretch and meditate as opposed to scrolling on the couch.

Fighting electronic addiction is difficult. So, like always, start small if you need to. Let's put the phone down, turn off the tv or computers, and see if we can stretch or meditate for twenty minutes. Without looking at the clock until you are done.

You got this! Enjoy all the cool things you will do with your reclaimed time this week!

25

Dance Party

> *Your homework for this section is to do a little dance when you have a moment.*

How to do your homework: While cleaning, cooking, at a stoplight, while shopping, wherever, put on some of your favorite music, take a quick moment to stop and dance. The most important thing is to dance your dance. Be free, be you, and enjoy the moment.

If you would like to, there are plenty of dance tutorials online. Regardless of the music you like. For most songs, you can go to YouTube and type the song you want followed by "dance fitness" and options will pop up.

How does this help you Be Better?

Dancing requires and improves our coordination, agility, balance, and self-awareness. All things needed to age both independently and actively. While dancing you need to be free, but also aware of how your body moves, body positioning, and how your body feels. Dancing is a fantastic way to keep our bodies active and limber.

Dance therapy is used to promote healing, well-being, and gain confidence. Dancing releases dopamine, serotonin, and endorphins which are neurotransmitters responsible for pleasure, mood, and euphoria, respectively. Dancing also releases the hormone oxytocin which increases the sense of trust, bonding, relaxation, memory, and love. The rise in these neurotransmitters and oxytocin leads to higher perceived levels of pleasure, mood, social connection, and relaxation. All while lowering stress and anxiety.

Moreover, dancing may lower the risk of dementia. In a study published in 2003 from the New England Journal of Medicine, researchers compared eleven exercise modalities. Of those studied, the only one to lower the participants' risk of dementia was dancing.

I got started in the fitness industry due to dance fitness classes. I was morbidly obese and desperate for a change. I started going to dance classes with a friend. I was nervous at first, what if I missed the moves, was uncoordinated, or tripped over my feet? What if I could not figure it out?

What I learned was, no one noticed or cared about what I was doing. They were too busy making sure they preformed the right steps, or got their workout, that they did not even notice me. It took me a few weeks, but eventually, I came out of my shell.

Several weeks later, I was on the stage alongside my instructors. I gained so much confidence. Less than two years later, an instructor mentored me so I could become an instructor myself. And now I get to encourage the people who come to all my classes.

I want to share my favorite story about this homework. I told my dance fitness class that their homework was to stop and dance at the stoplights on the way home. One of my favorite clients, who is in her sixties, and loves to jump and high kick, beamed when I gave this homework. The next week, she came to class all smiles. Telling the class that as she did the homework on her way home, a group of high school boys joined in and danced with her. And how happy it made her and them.

She encouraged them to dance their dance; and they encouraged my client in return. Just like all the people once encouraged me. And now, I want to encourage you to do the same.

So, what are you waiting for? Put on your favorite music and do a little dance!

26

Be Thankful

Your homework everyday this week is to find something you are thankful for.

How do you do your homework: Find a reason, big or small, to be thankful. You could be thankful for a sunny day, a good night's sleep, time spent with a loved one, a good parking space, or free time by yourself. It does not matter, just something you are thankful for.

You get bonus points if you can find something you are thankful for in a task you may not like. Examples of this in my life: Sometimes I may not want to exercise, but I am thankful I have a body that is capable of exercise. Sometimes I may not want to cook, but I am thankful I get to eat healthy food to better nourish my body. Sometimes I may not want to wash dishes (who does?), but I am thankful I have a dishwasher to assist with that chore. Somedays, the laundry feels never ending, but I am glad there are clothes to wash, a washing machine to do it, and the confidence I gain from wearing those clothes.

How does this help you Be Better?

Being thankful and grateful benefits your heart and soul.

When we practice gratitude, we shift our mindset of concentrating on the negatives of life to the more positive aspects. This helps release different neurotransmitters and hormones like oxytocin, dopamine, and serotonin known for boosting mood.

Oxytocin is the love hormone. It aids sleep, builds bonds, and lowers stress. Dopamine works as a natural pain reliever, leaving the body feeling better overall. Serotonin helps to regulate sleep, mood, and stress response. These hormones help ensure the quality and amount of sleep. Good sleep leads to better immunology response, digestion, and outlook on life.

Practicing thankfulness with our family, friends, and community strengthens those relationships and bonds. Thankfulness and gratitude are transferable. When we practice gratitude to those around us, we intrinsically feel good, but the people who receive it also feel good.

When my child was young, we would walk every morning to school. The mornings in Oregon are often cold and wet, and I admit I was not always excited to go.

But on our walks to and from school, my hand stayed warm intertwined in theirs. I had uninterrupted time to listen and talk with my child. To learn about their day, to make inside jokes. And though some mornings were harder than others, I was always thankful.

We no longer walk to school, but we find other ways to enjoy the time we have together, and considering those moments are much fewer, I am more thankful for them now.

It is important to recognize all the good that you encounter but also to understand that the good comes from outside of ourselves. We would not be where we are, who we are, or why we are, without the help of others.

Can you think of something that makes your life easier, for instance, your home? Have you thanked your home for providing safety and comfort? Have you shown your appreciation by taking good care and pride for it?

What else makes your life better? Take a moment to appreciate and give gratitude to that. Can you think of a task you may not like, but something in that task that helps you or brings you joy?

Can you think of anyone you are thankful for? Have you let them know that you appreciate them, and they have impacted you? Take a moment and really think about the things you are thankful for.

I am thankful for each one of you who have chosen to take the time out of your day to read this book, learn something new, and Be Better in the process.

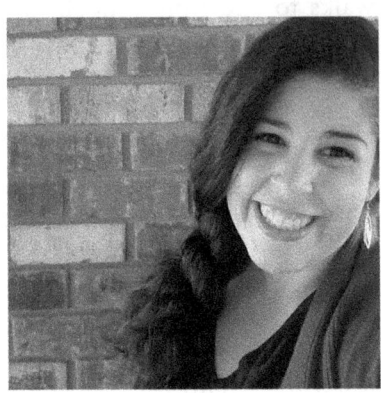

Jen's journey to being healthier came after a wake up call that she couldn't keep up with her one year old son. Determined to change that, she chose to make healthier habits, try new things, lose weight, and gain self confidence. While on that journey, Jen fell in love with group fitness classes and decided to make her passion her career. Over years, Jen developed her homework to help encourage clients to make healthier choices.

Outside of her fitness classes, Jen enjoys playing board games, painting, going on hikes, swimming, and dancing. She enjoys the nature of the wonderful Pacific Northwest, which she calls home. During the summers she can be found flying a kite and building sandcastles at the beach, or camping on the mountains.

Jen's biggest love, inspiration, and support come from her husband, Jonathan, and son, Jude.

www.ingramcontent.com/pod-product-compliance
Lightning Source LLC
Chambersburg PA
CBHW070519030426
42337CB00016B/2018